The Obesity Settle:

How To Defeat Nourishment Longings, Reduce Weight

And Pick Up Vitality

By

Mary J. Smith

Table of contents

Introduction

Obesity is a global public health issue with rising incidence and prevalence, expensive treatment options, and negative results. It has only been around for roughly a century as a disease with clear pathologic and pathophysiologic consequences. The word "obesity" did not enter the English language until the seventeenth century, and even then, it was only used in literature as a descriptor for excessive fatness or corpulence. The effects of obesity on quality of life started to be understood and documented in the eighteenth century, but it wasn't until the middle of the nineteenth century that it was acknowledged as a contributing factor to poor health, and only then were its morbid complications and increased mortality documented.

The exponential rise in obesity occurrence over the past 60 years, which prompted the World Health Organization to label it a global pandemic and a public health issue, has made this creeping medicalization of obesity worrying.

Obesity is a chronic condition, much like the other deadly illnesses (heart, vascular, and respiratory) that have become the bane of humanity over the same time. Since it is a chronic condition, its morbidity and mortality are due to the slow development of its comorbidities, such as diabetes, hypertension, and atherosclerosis. Contrary to other chronic diseases, it does not kill silently but instead manifests externally in the form of weight gain and increased girth, which is immediately noticeable to those who are affected by it. Therefore, as a public health issue, this outwardly apparent disease is simple to recognize, allowing a significant time to avert its effects.

At best, prevention is a difficult task, and problems are "a bomb waiting to be defused."

Obesity's earliest recorded occurrences date back at least 25 000 years. Obesity was considered an illness by Hippocrates in the Antique, but it was considered a sign of riches, power, and fertility throughout the Stone Age, Middle Ages, and 17th centuries. The Industrial Revolution saw the publication of the first scholarly studies on obesity. People had to contend with quackery and risky treatments like amphetamines that flooded the market during the 19th-century pharmacological treatment boom for obesity. The RYGB procedure is currently the gold standard in bariatric surgery, which was

 first performed in the 20th century.

One of the major issues facing public health today is the management of morbid obesity and associated comorbidities.

To learn how to avoid, control, and improve obesity, I just implore you to thoroughly read this book. Yes! The journey may be challenging but remain devoted to the goal. You can accomplish it.

Chapter One
Factors of Obesity

Being obese is the result of having too much bodily fat. One of the largest health issues around the globe is obesity.

A grouping of related illnesses, called metabolic

syndrome is linked to it. A few of these include an unhealthy blood lipid profile, elevated blood pressure, and high blood sugar. Compared to people whose weight is within a normal range, those with metabolic syndrome have a significantly increased risk of developing heart disease and type 2 diabetes.

The causes of obesity and possible prevention or treatment strategies have been the subject of a lot of research over the past few decades.

A lot of people seem to have the idea that a lack of willpower is what prompts weight gain and obesity. That's not accurate.

Notwithstanding the fact that eating habits and way of life choices account for the whole excess weight problem, some people have difficulty in this area. The issue is that a variety of biotic factors, including heredity and hormones, contribute to overeating. Some folks simply tend to gain weight.

Certainly, individuals can modify their way of life and behavior to compensate for the disadvantages of congenital traits. Persistence, willpower, and devotion are the keys to making a lifestyle change.

However, it is facile to state that behavior is merely the aftermath of willpower.

They don't consider all the other elements that eventually influence people's actions and timing. A recent study on adult obesity in America took place in the year 2017–18. The prevalence increased from 30.5% in 1999–2000 to 42.5%. The prevalence of class III obesity increased from 4.7% to 9.2% throughout that time, nearly doubling. America had a 19.3% childhood obesity rate from 2017 to 2018.

Over the past 50 years, the global obesity rate has tripled. Obesity has been particularly pronounced in impoverished nations where malnutrition is widespread. Now more people in these neighborhoods have access to higher-calorie, lower-nutritional foods. In many nations, dietary deficiency and obesity are now excessively concurrent conditions. Despite government efforts to inform citizens of the need for adopting healthy lifestyles, more adults and children are being diagnosed with obesity. Even though obesity has many origins, Americans should be concerned about its effects on society. In addition to lowering society's productivity, rising obesity rates also have other negative effects, but it will also encourage the government to set aside more money to cover the costs of treating diseases connected to fat.

Given that obesity is a significant issue in American culture and that it has the potential to negatively impact both health outcomes and economic productivity, people need to start taking it more seriously.

Because there are numerous contributing factors to obesity, there must be a variety of targets and treatments to address each one. Here are 15 factors, many of which have nothing to do with willpower, that are major contributors to weight gain, obesity, and metabolic disease.

Genetics

There is a great congenital trait component to obesity. Compared to youngsters of slim parents, youngsters of obese parents are considerably more expected to be obese.

However, the aforementioned does not suggest that obesity is totally predictable.

Which congenital traits are manifested and which aren't can exceedingly depend on what you consume.

When non-industrialized countries select normal Western food, obesity rates magnify rapidly in such societies. Their genes did not significantly modify them; rather, the signals sent to their genes by their environment and the environment itself did. In simple terms, genetic factors do impact your chances of gaining weight. This is very well illustrated by studies on identical twins.

Availability of Food

Food availability, which has expanded significantly over the past few centuries, is another element that has a significant impact on people's waistlines. Food, especially fast food, is widely available today. In stores, appealing items are displayed in areas where you are most likely to see them.

Another issue is that, especially in America, unhealthy, whole meals are frequently more affordable.

Some folks, especially those who live in less affluent areas, don't even have access to real food options like fresh fruits and vegetables. These communities only have convenience stores that sell beverages, candies, and processed packaged junk food. If there is no choice, how can it be a matter of choice?

Insulin

One of the many things that insulin controls is how much energy is stored.

Its job includes instructing fat cells to store fat and retain any fat they already contain. Many overweight and obese people's Western diets encourage insulin resistance. As a result, the body's insulin levels rise throughout, causing energy to be stored in fat cells as opposed to being used.

Although there is debate regarding insulin's relationship to obesity, numerous research point to a causal relationship between elevated insulin levels and the emergence of obesity. Reducing your diet to simple or refined carbs while increasing your intake of fiber is one of the best methods to lower your insulin. Without the need for portion control or calorie tracking, this typically results in a spontaneous decrease in caloric intake and uncomplicated weight loss.

Violent Marketing

Marketers for manufacturers of junk food are quite aggressive. Sometimes they try to promote extremely unhealthy products as healthy ones, which is an unethical technique. These businesses also make false statements. Even worse, they specifically target youngsters with their marketing.

Children are becoming obese, diabetic, and hooked to junk food in modern society before they are mature enough to make these kinds of decisions for themselves.

Food Dependence

Your brain's reward regions are activated by a lot of high-fat, sugar-sweetened junk food. People who consume more of these foods experience increased food cravings because of the foods' high sugar content. These meals are frequently contrasted with drugs that are frequently abused, such as alcohol, cocaine, nicotine, and cannabis.

Junk food addiction can develop in those who are vulnerable. Similar to how those who struggle with alcohol addiction lose control over their drinking, these people also lose control over their eating.

Addiction is a complicated problem that can be very challenging to resolve.

When you get dependent on something, you lose your freedom of choice and your brain's biochemistry takes control. Some individuals have significant food dependencies or strong desire for food. This is particularly true of junk foods high in fat and sugar that activate the brain's reward regions.

Particular Drugs

As a side effect, several medicinal medicines might make you gain weight.

For instance, antidepressants have been associated with gradual weight gain.

Antipsychotic drugs and medications for diabetes are more examples. These medications do not weaken your willpower. They change how your body and brain work, slowing down or speeding up your metabolism.

There are several medications, such as some corticosteroids, that can also make you gain weight.

Resistance to leptin

Another hormone that has a significant impact on obesity is leptin. It is produced by fat cells, and as fat mass increases, blood levels rise. Leptin levels are hence particularly high in obese individuals.

High leptin levels are associated with decreased appetite in healthy individuals. It should communicate to your brain how much fat you have when it's functioning properly. Leptin is not functioning properly in many obese persons because, for unknown reasons, it cannot penetrate the blood-brain barrier.

Leptin resistance is a condition that is thought to be a major contributor to the pathophysiology of obesity.

Artificial junk food

Foods that have undergone extensive processing typically only contain refined components and additives.

These goods are made to be inexpensive, durable, and difficult to resist due to their incredible flavor. Food producers aim to boost sales by making products as tasty as possible. However, they also encourage overeating.

Today's processed foods tend to have very little in common with whole foods. These items are carefully crafted and made to hook consumers.

Sugar

It is possible that added sweetening is the worst element of the modern diet.

That's because consuming too much sugar alters your body's biochemistry and hormones. In turn, this results in a weight increase.

Half of the added sugar is glucose and half is fructose. Foods like starch can provide people with glucose, but added sugar is where most fructose is found.

These foods account for 90% of the refined sugars we consume, which contributes to obesity and overweight, which in turn cause various health problems. Increased insulin levels and insulin resistance may result from consuming too much sugar. Additionally, it does not stimulate satiety the same way that glucose does.

Energy is stored in the body, due to sugar intake which eventually leads to obesity.

Environment

The environment we reside has an importance on our propensity to keep a healthy weight. For instance:

It is challenging for people to be physically active when there are no nearby parks, sidewalks, or reasonably priced gyms.

Americans' calorie consumption rises as a result of oversized meal portions, necessitating even more exercise to maintain a healthy weight.

Some folks lack access to grocery stores that offer reasonably priced healthful foods, like fresh fruits and vegetables.

People are influenced by food advertising to purchase unhealthy items like sugary drinks and high-fat snacks.

Sleep

People spend a significant amount of time using electronic devices, including lights and televisions, as well as the Internet, video games, and other forms of entertainment. The cell phone for instance affects how much rest individuals are getting. Additionally, studies have shown that people are more likely to be overweight or obese the less sleep they get. This is partly because hormones generated when you sleep help regulate your appetite and how much energy your body uses. Additionally, it is linked to a higher incidence of blood pressure, diabetes, and pain issues.

Stress and emotional factors

When they are bored, irritated, disturbed, or stressed, some people eat more than normal. Short-term stress results in the brain producing the hormone corticotrophin-releasing hormone, which suppresses hunger. As part of the fight-or-flight response, impulses given to the adrenal glands during times of stress cause them to produce adrenalin, which momentarily suppresses the urge to eat.

On the other hand, persistent stress results in the release of the hormone cortisol. If the stress does not subside, the hormone cortisol and the person's hunger both remain elevated. We all know that overeating results in weight gain.

False information

People are ignorant about diet and health all around the world.

There are several causes for this, but the issue is mostly influenced by the sources of information that people use. For instance, a lot of websites disseminate false or outright misleading advice regarding nutrition and health.

The findings of scientific studies are regularly taken out of context in some news outlets, and they are sometimes oversimplified or misinterpreted. Some material may simply be out-of-date or based on unproven theories.

As well, food businesses are involved. Some advertise useless things, like weight loss supplements. Strategies for losing weight that is based on erroneous information can impede your progress. It's crucial to make wise source selections.

 A bad diet

Obesity does not develop suddenly. It gradually manifests over time as a result of poor dietary habits and lifestyle decisions, including: consuming a lot of processed or fast food that is heavy in fat and sugar and drinking excessive amounts of alcohol. Alcohol has a lot of calories, and heavy drinkers frequently overindulge in eating out. In a restaurant, you might be tempted to order a starter or dessert as well, and the food might be higher in fat and sugar. If your friends or family are consuming excessive amounts of sugary beverages, such as soft drinks and fruit juice, while also consuming enormous servings of food, you could feel more inclined to do the same. If you're feeling down or unmotivated, you might eat to cheer yourself up. Eating disorders frequently run in families.

When you're young, you could pick up unhealthy eating habits from your parents that you carry into adulthood.

Pregnancy

It's normal to gain weight while pregnant. Some ladies find it very hard to reduce this weight after delivery. This weight increase could result in obesity later on.

Chapter Two
The classifications or types of obesity

Body mass index (BMI) is a straightforward measure of weight to height that is frequently used to categorize adults as overweight and obese. By dividing an individual's weight in kilograms by the square of his or her height in meters (kg/m2) BMI can be determined.

Adults

According to the WHO, an adult is considered overweight if their BMI is larger than or equal to 25, and obese if their BMI is greater than or equal to 30.

The most helpful population-level indicator of overweight and obesity is BMI because it is applicable to individuals of all sexes and ages.

But because it might not equate to the same level of fatness in various people, it should only be used as a general reference

Children

Children under the age of five:

Obesity is defined as weight-for-height that is more than three standard deviations above the WHO Child Growth Standards median and is larger than 2 standard deviations above overweight.

Obesity is frequently identified using the body mass index (BMI).

Asians with a BMI of 23 or higher may be more susceptible to health issues.

The BMI presents a reliable approximation of body fat for the majority of people. Body

Mass Index does not, however, exactly measure body fat, hence some individuals, such as muscular athletes, may have a BMI that falls into the category of obesity despite having normal levels of body fat.

Many physicians additionally take an outpatient's waist measurement to boost treatment planning. Weight-related health problems are more likely in men with a waist circumference over 40 inches (102 centimeters) and in women with a waist measurement over 35 inches (89 centimeters) (89 centimeters).

Due to its high incidence, increased risk of various diseases, and shorter lifespan, obesity is a global public health issue. As with adipocyte metabolism, it results from a complex combination of genetic, lifestyle, dietary habits, energy expenditure, nutritional, and metabolic factors.

The idea that adipose tissue and skeletal muscle play a role in lipid and glucose metabolism has supplanted the common understanding that these tissues serve as energy storage because of the abundance of bioactive proteins referred to as adipokines and myokines that are produced and linked to some cardiovascular risk factors influences of obesity.

Furthermore, pro-inflammatory cytokines released by numerous cell types that also appear to be important regulators of adipose tissue metabolism are closely linked to low-grade systemic inflammation, which in turn is closely associated with obesity and glucose metabolism. The biggest drawback of any method that limits the diagnosis of obesity to the amount of weight and circumference gain while ignoring changes in body composition such as an increase in body fat percentage and a decrease in lean body mass is that it ignores the effects of adiposity on physiological and metabolic processes that lead to higher rates of morbidity and mortality. It is crucial to categorize obesity based on body fat composition and distribution rather than just the rise in body weight because of the endocrine and inflammatory roles played by adipose tissue. To conveniently approximate body fat percentage and classify people, the body mass index (BMI), which is a ratio of weight to the square of height (kg/m2) of a subject, introduces a significant mistake and misclassification. Underweight (BMI 18.5 kg/m2), normal weight (BMI 18.5-24.9 kg/m2), class I obesity - overweight (BMI 25.0-29.9 kg/m2), class II obesity - obesity (BMI 30.0-39.9 kg/m2), and class III obesity - extreme obesity (BMI > 40 kg/m2) are the five classifications according to BMI.

Obesity and being overweight are associated with a greater risk of 13 different types of cancer.

These tumors consist of—

Esophageal adenocarcinoma.

Breast (for ladies who have gone through menopause).

rectum and colon.

Uterus.

Gallbladder.

upper abdomen

Kidneys.

Liver.

Ovaries.

Pancreas.

Thyroid.

Meningioma (a type of brain cancer).

Several myelomas.

Type 2 diabetes, cardiovascular disease, hypertension, high cholesterol, stroke, non-alcoholic fatty liver disease, arthritis, eating disorders like bulimia, and mental health conditions like depression and low self-esteem are some of the other health effects of obesity that have been described.

Obesity symptoms and signs

Obesity symptoms extend beyond having too much body fat. Someone who is obese may experience skin issues, breathing difficulties, trouble sleeping, and other issues.

You may be more susceptible to certain diseases and disorders if you experience certain symptoms. These can occasionally be fatal or life-threatening.

Common Obesity Symptoms in Adults

Adult obesity symptoms frequently include:

Extra body fat, especially at the waist

Breathing difficulty

More perspiration than usual

Snoring

Difficulty sleeping

Skin issues led by moisture buildup in the folds

Difficulty in carrying out easy physical activities that were no trouble before you put on weight

Mild to extreme fatigue
Excruciating pain especially in the joints and back
Mental health problems include low self-esteem, depression, shame, and social isolation.

Chapter Three
The calorie puzzle (Recognizing Calories)

Calories from various food sources help people lose weight more than calories from other sources. Calorie intake has no difference in terms of weight loss.

Do you believe the calories from fat, carbs, and protein vary?

No matter what food source it comes from, a calorie is always a calorie. You still consume 100 calories whether you eat 100 calories of yogurt or 100 calories of candy. Although the body typically burns calories from carbohydrates first, followed by calories from protein, and then calories from fat, many widely adopted diets have placed more emphasis on limiting the quantity of fat, carbohydrate, or protein consumed than on urging people to pay attention to their overall calorie intake.

Recognizing calories

Calories are a measurement of the amount of energy found in food and

beverages. Our bodies retain extra calories as body fat when we consume more than we burn off through food and drink. Over time, we might gain weight if this keeps happening. A typical male needs about 2,500 kcal (10,500 kJ) each day to keep fine body weight.

For a typical woman, that translates to around 2,000 kcal (8,400 kJ) each day.

In addition to age and size, active work

levels can also have an impact on these results.

Using the weight record (BMI) calculator, you can determine your healthy weight.

Your basic caloric admission should be calculated first.

Do this by multiplying your current weight by 10. For instance, 180 pounds multiplied by 10 equals 1,800.

Calories at Base = 1,800

The next thing you should consider is how active you are. You must consume more calories if you are more active, right? Senses well. You should therefore multiply your present weight by 2, 3, or 5 depending on your degree of activity. Use two if you are not engaged. Use three if you are a fairly active person. Use five if you're highly active. Suppose we have a moderate level of activity: 180 X 3 = 540.

calories from activity = 540

To determine how many calories you must consume each day to maintain your current weight, add your exercise calories to your base calories. 1,800 + 540 = 2,340.

Calories for maintenance: 2,340

An exception to this computation is that if you are over 50, deduct 10% from your maintenance calories. 2,340 - 234 = 2,106

Your Maintenance Calories if you are over 50 are 2,106

Let's find out how many calories you need every day if you want to lose weight. Since 3,500 calories make up one pound of body weight, you must cut 500 calories from your daily diet to lose one pound every week. Get it?

But I must warn you to never consume less than 1,200 calories each day. Your body needs a specific quantity of energy each day to function properly. Many people are unaware of how many calories they consume daily in alcohol. You can track your current calorie intake using a few free web tools. You may determine how far you are from your target by knowing approximately how many calories you are now consuming.

From there, you can start selecting foods to reduce the number of calories you eat each day. Cut back on your portion sizes by, for instance, giving up your afternoon coffee, selecting healthier snacks, drinking more water in place of sugary juices and drinks, and cutting back on your afternoon coffee. Be careful not to change things too significantly as you make these adjustments. Pace and consistency are the keys to winning the race. If you dramatically reduce your calorie intake, you run the risk of binging as a result of being overly hungry. Try to implement one or two good adjustments each day.

On another thought, you can get around this by exercising more if you feel like the number calculated above is too low for you and you just can't give those calories up. By stating that we were moderately active, we were able to calculate the values above.

Let's imagine you started an exercise program that qualifies you as more active. The results of your numbers are as follows…

Calories at Base Level: 180 x 10 = 1,800

180 × 5 (highly active) calories equal 900.

Calories for maintenance: 1,800 + 900 = 2,700

Calories Needed to Lose Weight: 2,700 − 500 = 2,200

You now have a whopping 360 calories to work with! To burn this many calories, for instance, you would need to jog for around 30 minutes at a pace of 10 minutes per mile.

Balance of calories and energy

Our bodies require the right amount of energy to continue functioning and to ensure that our organs are operating appropriately. By eating and drinking, we provide our bodies with energy. However, our bodies expend that energy through our daily activities.

The energy we put into our bodies must match the energy we use during regular biological processes and physical activity to maintain a stable weight. A key element of a balanced diet is striking a balance between the energy you put into your body and the energy you expend. Take, for example, we use up more energy when we engage in more physical activities. Do not be concerned if you consume too much energy in one day. In the following days, just make an effort to consume less energy.

Examining the number of calories in food

Realizing the calorie content of food and drink can assist with guaranteeing you're not polishing off something over the top.

The calorie content of many shop-purchased food sources is expressed on the bundling as a feature of the nourishment name. This data will show up under the "Energy" heading.

The calorie content is much of the time given in kcals, which is short for kilocalories, and in kJ, which is short for kilojoules. A kilocalorie is a different way to say what's generally called a calorie, so 1,000 calories will be composed of 1,000kcals.

Kilojoules are the metric estimation of calories. To find the energy content in kilojoules, duplicate the calorie figure by 4.2. You may compare the caloric content of various products by reading the label, which will typically state how many calories are present in 100 grams or 100 milliliters of the meal or drink.

Many labels will likewise express the number of calories in a single piece of food. In any case, recollect that the producer's concept of one portion may not be equivalent to yours, so there could be more calories in the piece you serve yourself. You may evaluate how a specific food fits into your daily calorie intake using the calorie information.

Calories countermeasures

There's an extensive variety of online calorie counters for PCs and cell phones. A considerable lot of these can be downloaded and utilized for nothing.

The NHS can't confirm their information, yet they can be useful in checking your calories by recording all of the food you eat in a day. A few eateries put calorie data on their menus, so you can likewise check the calorie content of food varieties while eating out. Calories ought to be given per segment or per feast.

Using up calories

How many calories individuals use by doing a specific actual work fluctuates, contingent upon the scope of variables, including size and age. The more energetically you do an action, the more calories you'll utilize.

For instance, quick strolling will consume a larger number of calories than strolling at a moderate speed.

Assuming you're putting on weight, it could mean you have been consistently eating and drinking a greater number of calories than you have been utilizing. To get thinner, you want to utilize more energy than you consume and proceed with this throughout some undefined time frame.

Become acclimated to counting calories

The best methodology is to join diet changes with expanded active work.

How do competitive eaters consume so much food while maintaining their physique?

This is because when you eat that much food your stomach can't process its majority. It isn't transformed into calories. Assuming you put that much food in your stomach you won't have sufficient stomach corrosive to manage it.

Individuals say "I have an elevated capacity to burn calories" No! that is off-base. They are regularly eating excessively because they are so restless, or their stomach-related framework may not fully function since they don't expend enough energy triggering the parasympathetic framework, so they are not processing a lot of what they are consuming. Then, on their off days, they exercise and consume low- or no-calorie meal options.

Chapter Four
Nutrition and Diet

Trans Fats, colorants, preservatives, and other additives added to previously unexistent foods only to add flavor result in calories. Most people are unaware of how important it is for the human body to have a good balance of all the nutrients and chemical elements. Most people give their diet of fruits and vegetables and vitamin C very little thought.

The majority of individuals consume excessive calories from poor-quality foods, which causes weight gain, but they do not consume nearly enough micronutrients to meet their body's needs. In America, the majority of people consume excessive amounts of hydrogenated oils, trans fats, high-fructose corn syrup, artificial sweeteners, preservatives, and other synthetic substances.

The majority of Americans are short in nutrients that support health and vitality, including fruits, vitamins, and high-protein foods like pork and fish. It's a well-known fact that how many calories individuals eat and drink straightforwardly affects their weight: Consume the very number of calories that the body consumes over the long haul, and weight stays stable. Consume more than the body expends, weight increases. Less, weight goes down. However, what might be said about the kind of calories: Does it matter if they originate from certain foods, such as fat, protein, or carbohydrates? Certain food varieties: entire grains or potato chips? Certain weight control plans: the Mediterranean eating routine or the "Twinkie" diet? Furthermore, shouldn't something be said about when or where individuals consume their calories: Does having breakfast make it more straightforward to control weight? Does eating at drive-through joints make it harder? There's an adequate exploration of food sources and diet designs that safeguard against coronary illness, stroke, diabetes, and other constant circumstances. Fortunately a considerable lot of the food sources that assist with forestalling sickness likewise appear to assist with weight control; food sources like entire grains, fruits, vegetables, and nuts. What's more, a significant number of food sources that increase sickness risk like; refined grains and sweet beverages are likewise considered weight gain. According to conventional knowledge, eating less and exercising more is the ideal strategy for weight management because calories come from all sources, regardless of their source.

However, rising research proposes that a few food varieties and eating examples might make it simpler to hold calories within proper limits, while others might make individuals bound to consume more.

This audits the exploration of dietary admission and weight control, featuring diet methodologies that assist with forestalling persistent infection.

Which is more vital for controlling weight: carbohydrates, protein, or fat?

The percentage of calories from fat, protein, and carbohydrates in a regulated diet does not appear to affect how much weight a person loses. A higher protein, lower carbohydrate diet may have some advantages in studies where participants are free to pick what they consume. However, the quality and food sources of these nutrients matter more for the prevention of chronic diseases than their relative amounts in the diet. The most recent research also indicates that the same diet quality message applies to weight management.

Food Fat and Body weight

Low-fat diets have long been hailed as the secret to healthy weight loss and overall wellness.

But the proof simply isn't there:

In the past 30 years, Americans' diets have contained fewer calories from fat, but obesity rates have increased dramatically.

Following a low-fat diet does not make it any simpler to lose weight than following a moderate- or high-fat diet, according to carefully conducted research trials.

In reality, study participants on moderate- or high-fat diets lose the same amount of weight—and in some studies, even a little more—as those on low-fat diets.

Low-fat diets don't seem to have any unique advantages when it comes to disease prevention.

Low-fat diets can be problematic since they frequently contain large amounts of carbohydrates, particularly those from foods that digest quickly, like white rice and bread. Furthermore, eating a lot of these items raises your chance of developing diabetes, heart disease, and weight gain. There is some evidence that the type of fat a person consumes may be just as crucial for weight control as it is for good health. Increased consumption of unhealthy fats—trans fats, especially, but also saturated fats—was linked to weight gain in the Nurses' Health Study, which monitored 42,000 middle-aged and older women for eight years. However, increased consumption of healthy fats—monounsaturated and polyunsaturated fat—was not.

Weight and protein

Although more so in short-term research, higher protein diets do appear to offer some advantages for weight loss; but, in longer-term studies, high-protein diets appear to perform similarly well as other types of diets. It is challenging to distinguish the health benefits of eating a lot of protein from those of eating more fat or less carbohydrate because high-protein diets tend to be low in carbohydrates and high in fat. However, there are a few reasons why consuming more calories from protein might aid in weight management:

Higher satiety: People will quite often feel more full, on fewer calories, in the wake of eating protein than they do after eating starch or fat.

More thermogenic impact: Protein has a higher thermic effect than other macronutrients since it requires more energy to process and store than other foods.

Further developed body piece: Lean muscle retention appears to be aided by protein consumption during weight reduction, which can also increase the energy expended side of the energy balance equation.

Blood lipid profiles and other metabolic indicators are improved by higher protein, and reduced carbohydrate diets, so they might assist with forestalling heart disease and diabetes. Be that as it may, some high-protein food varieties are more nutritious than others: High admissions of red meat and flavored meat are related to an expanded risk of heart disease, diabetes, and stomach cancerous growth.

Replace red and flavored meat with nuts, legumes, fish, or chicken to reduce your chance of developing diabetes and heart disease. What's more, this diet technique might assist with weight control, as well, as indicated by a new report from the Harvard School of Public Health. Analysts followed the eating routine and way of life propensities of 120,000 people for as long as 20 years, seeing how little changes added to weight gain over the long run. Individuals who ate more red and flavored meat throughout the review put on more weight-about a pound extra every four years. Individuals who ate more nuts throughout the review put on less weight-about a half pound less every four years.

Weight and carbohydrate

Lower carb, higher protein diets might have some weight reduction benefits temporarily. However with regards to forestalling weight gain and constant infection, carb quality is considerably more significant than sugar amount. White rice, white bread, white pasta, processed morning cereals, and similar items manufactured with milled, refined grains are high in quickly absorbed carbohydrates. Potatoes and sweet beverages are as well. They have a high glycemic load, which is the medical word for this, as well as a high glycemic index. Such food sources cause quick and angry expansions in glucose and insulin that, temporarily, can make hunger spike and can prompt gorging, and over the long haul, raise the chance of developing diabetes, heart disease, and weight gain.

As an illustration, in the eating routine and way of life change study, individuals who expanded their intakes of refined grains and sweet beverages,potatoes, potato chips and french fries, put on more weight, an extra 3.4, 1.3, 1.0, and 0.6 pounds like every four years, separately. Individuals who diminished their admission of these food sources put on less weight.

Certain meals that affect how easy or difficult it is to control weight

There is mounting evidence that some meal selections may aid with weight management.

Fruits and vegetables, whole grains, and weight

Fruits and Vegetables

Fruits and vegetables have an extremely advantageous nutritional makeup.

They are a recommended dietary alternative for weight loss because they are low in calories and abundant in essential elements. Vegetables were typically ingested in between meals that were well-balanced whereas fruits are typically consumed as part of a wholesome or complete meal.

The weight-control evidence for whole grains is stronger than it is for fruits and vegetables. The most recent evidence comes from a diet and lifestyle change study conducted by the Harvard School of Public Health. Participants who consumed more whole grains, whole fruits (instead of fruit juice), and vegetables throughout the 20-year study, respectively, gained less weight, losing 0.4, 0.5, and 0.2 pounds every four years.

Naturally, the calories from entire grains, fruits, and veggies remain. People who consume more of these items tend to consume fewer calories from other foods, which is probably what is happening. Since fiber slows digestion and helps to reduce appetite, it may be a fiber that is responsible for these meals' positive effects on weight control. In addition to being high in water, fruits and vegetables may help people feel fuller with fewer calories.

Whole grains

Such as whole wheat, brown rice, barley, and others—are metabolized more slowly than refined grains, especially in their less-processed forms. They, therefore, have a milder impact on insulin and blood sugar, which might aid in preventing hunger. The majority of fruits and vegetables share this trait.

There are numerous advantages to eating these "low carb" meals for illness prevention, and there is evidence that they can also aid in weight loss.

Weight and Nuts

Nuts were formerly shunned by dieters because they contain a lot of calories in a small amount and are high in fat. As it turns out, studies show that eating nuts does not result in weight gain and may even aid in weight management. This may be because nuts are high in protein and fiber, both of which may make people feel fuller and more satiety-inducing and prevent overeating. Another reason to include nuts in a healthy diet is that people who consume them frequently have a lower risk of developing heart disease or dying from it than those who consume them infrequently.

Weight and Dairy

Based largely on the results of short-term research it funded, the U.S. dairy industry has aggressively promoted the benefits of milk and other dairy products for weight loss. However, a recent analysis of over 50 randomized trials reveals less support for the idea that consuming plenty of dairy products or calcium promotes weight loss. Similar to this, the majority of long-term follow-up studies have not discovered that dairy or calcium prevent weight growth, and one study in adolescents discovered a link between excessive milk intake and an elevated body mass index. One exception is the most current dietary and lifestyle modification study from the Harvard School of Public Health, which discovered that those who increased their yogurt intake gained less weight; however, increases in milk and cheese intake did not appear to promote either weight loss or gain.

Yogurt's helpful bacteria may affect how you manage your weight, but more research is required.

Weight and Sugar-Sweetened Beverages

There is strong evidence to support the claim that sugary beverages raise the risk of weight gain, obesity, and diabetes: Clear correlations between the consumption of soft drinks and increased calorie intake and body weight were observed in a comprehensive review and meta-analysis of 88 research.

According to a more recent meta-analysis, the body mass index rises by 0.08 units for every additional 12-ounce serving of sugary beverage ingested daily in children and adolescents. According to a second meta-study, those who frequently drink sugary drinks had a 26% higher chance of acquiring type 2 diabetes than those who do not often use these drinks. A growing body of research also points to an increased risk of heart disease with excessive sugar beverage use.

Like refined grains and potatoes, sweet refreshments are high in quickly processed carbs. The research proposes that people don't eat less to make up for the extra calories when carbohydrate is given to them in liquid form rather than solid form since it doesn't make them feel as satisfied.

Given that both adults and children are consuming increasing amounts of sugary beverages, the following facts are concerning: In the United States, sugared beverages made up around 4% of daily caloric consumption in the 1970s but made up about 9% of calories in 2001. According to the most recent statistics, fifty percent of Americans eat some kind of sugary beverage on any given day, twenty-five percent consume at least 200 calories from sugary drinks, and five percent consume at least 567 calories, which is the same as four cans of sugary soda.

The good news is that research on both children and adults has demonstrated that reducing the use of sugar-sweetened beverages can result in weight loss. Sugary beverages have emerged as a key focus of attempts to fight obesity, bringing up the possibility of legislative measures like soda taxes.

Weight and fruit juice

It's critical to take note that fruit juices are not a preferable choice for weight management over sugar-improved refreshments. Fruit juices, even those that are 100 percent fruit juice and include no additional sugar, are just as high in sugar and calories per ounce as sugary drinks. So it's nothing unexpected that a new Harvard School of Public Health review, which followed the eating regimen and way of life propensities for 120,000 people for as long as 20 years, found that individuals who expanded their admission of fruits juice put on more weight after some time than individuals who didn't. Children and adults should limit their consumption of fruit juice to no more than one small glass per day, if at all, according to pediatricians and public health activists.

Weight and Alcoholic Liquor
Even though most liquors have a larger number of calories per ounce than sugar-improved refreshments, there's no obvious proof that moderate drinking adds to weight gain.

While the new eating routine and way of life change investigation discovered that individuals who expanded their liquor consumption put on more weight after some time, the results differed depending on the type of alcohol consumed.

Light-to-moderate drinkers gained less weight than nondrinkers over time in the majority of prior prospective studies, or there was no difference between the two groups' weight growth over time.

Chapter Five
Pregnancy and Obesity

Everyone agrees that pregnancy is the time when one or more offspring grows (gestates) inside a woman's womb. When the components of a vigorous sperm and a viable ovum, or egg, combine, a new individual is born.

Pregnancy-related weight gain varies widely.

The majority of weight gained by pregnant women, between 10kg and 12.5kg (22lb to 28lb), occurs after week 20.

The growth of your baby is largely to blame for the extra weight, but your body will also be storing fat in preparation for producing breast milk once your baby is born.

Although the majority of the weight growth will occur in the second and third trimesters, the first 12 weeks of pregnancy will see some early weight gain.

In reality, weight gain during the first trimester ranges from 1 to 4 pounds on average, but it might fluctuate.

How much weight should a pregnant woman gain?

You may have heard that while you're pregnant, you should gain 25 to 35 pounds. However, that range only applies to those who were "normal weight" before becoming pregnant according to their body mass index (BMI).

You will slowly put on weight as your baby grows. The amount of weight you gain can have an impact on your health and the health of your unborn child. For example, too much weight gain can increase your risk of gestational diabetes.

When pregnant, a lady who was of average weight before becoming pregnant should put on 25 to 35 pounds. Underweight ladies need to acquire between 28 and 40 pounds. Additionally, obese women might only need to put on 15 to 25 pounds during pregnancy.

Generally speaking, you should gain 1 pound each week for the remainder of your pregnancy and 2 to 4 pounds for the first three months of your pregnancy. You should put on 35 to 45 pounds throughout pregnancy if you're having twins. After the typical weight growth in the first three months, this would be an average of 1½ pounds per week.

When you're expecting twins, it's extremely crucial to gain the correct amount of weight because your weight impacts the weight of the infants. Additionally, twins' health depends on their birth weight being higher because they frequently arrive earlier than expected. You can require between 3,000 and 3,500 calories per day when having twins. The recommended weight increase for twins during pregnancy is as follows:

Weight loss: 50 to 62 pounds
Weight range: 37 to 54 pounds
 Overweight: 31 to 50 pounds
Obese: 25 to 42 pounds

Women, however, experience this differently.

An analysis of pregnancy weight

Ever wonder where pregnancy weight disappears to?

The truth is that even while it may seem like everything is in your stomach, it is not. Here is

a rough breakdown of a 30-pound pregnancy weight gain:
7.5-pound infant
1.5 pounds of placenta
2 pounds of amniotic fluid
2 pounds of uterine hypertrophy
2 pounds of maternal breast tissue
The blood volume in the mother: 4 pounds
4 pounds of fluids in the maternal tissue
7 pounds of maternal fat storage

To have a healthy pregnancy and infant, as well as to get your body ready for breastfeeding if you intend to do so, you need to put on weight in each of these regions.

Weight growth in the first trimester

Your kid is still quite small, so you might only need to gain 2 to 4 pounds in total. You can gain less or perhaps lose a little weight if you have morning sickness. It's ok; over the next six months, you can lose those extra pounds.

On the other side, you can put on a little bit of extra weight during the first trimester if you have strong pregnancy cravings. In any case, your practitioner will assist you in developing a strategy for the next two.

Weight growth in the second trimester

Between weeks 12 and 16 of pregnancy, morning sickness typically subsides just as your baby begins to grow seriously. Your pregnancy weight gain should ideally increase throughout the second trimester so that you gain a total of 12 to 14 pounds.

Weight growth in the third trimester

While your weight growth may start to taper off for a net gain of about 8 to 10 pounds, the baby's weight gain will accelerate in the final few months of your pregnancy. While finding room for meals can be challenging throughout the ninth month due to ever-tighter abdominal space, some women find their weight maintains steady or even decreases during this time. If you shed a few pounds near the conclusion of your pregnancy, that's quite normal.

Remember that these are averages rather than strict formulas.

You'll experience periods where you're constantly hungry and weeks were eating a lot of anything will make your stomach spin.

You're on the correct track if your overall pregnancy weight gain is within range and you're increasing at a rate that makes sense.

What is a typical pregnancy weight gain?

Your pre-pregnancy weight will determine how much weight you gain during your pregnancy.

Calculate your pre-pregnancy body mass index first before determining how much weight you should acquire (BMI). The way to calculate this is stated below:

the square of your height divided by the number of kgs you weighed before becoming pregnant (in meters).

Therefore, 68 / 1.7 x 1.7 = 23.5 would be your BMI if you were 1.7m tall and 68kg.

To calculate your BMI before becoming pregnant, use the BMI calculator.

You were in the healthy weight range before being pregnant if your BMI was between 18.5 and 24.9, and you should ideally gain between 11.5 and 16 kg: 1 to 1.5 kg during the first three months, then 1.5 to 2 kg each month until you give birth.

What is the impact of being overweight on a woman's ability to conceive?

Being overweight typically has no impact on a woman's ability to conceive. Obesity, as opposed to being overweight, can lower your chances of getting pregnant. The reason for this is that being overweight may interfere with your hormones and inhibit your ovaries from releasing an egg (ovulation). The same type of issue might arise from being underweight.

Additionally, some research indicates that being obese may increase your risk of miscarriage or pregnancy problems.

However, a lot of fat people have no trouble getting pregnant and don't have these health problems.

Acquiring a lot of weight

Putting on an excess weight can influence your well-being and increment your circulatory strain.

Be that as it may, pregnancy isn't an ideal opportunity to deprive oneself of food, as it might hurt the well-being of the unborn child. You should eat strongly.

Acquiring an excess of weight can build your risk of complexities.

These include:

1. Gestational diabetes: Producing gestational diabetes during pregnancy increases the likelihood of having a large-framed baby since it is brought on by having too much glucose (sugar) in the blood during pregnancy.
2. Pre-eclampsia: Although most cases are mild and cause no problems, they can be serious. The onset of pre-eclampsia may be indicated by an increase in blood pressure.
3. Cesarean section: A cesarean section is a medical procedure that involves cutting through the mother's abdominal wall to deliver the baby.
4. Macrosomia: The term "macrosomic" refers to a fetus that weighs more than 4000–4500 grams (or 9–10 pounds). A newborn who was overweight at birth is

referred to as having macrosomia.

5. Stillbirth: A stillbirth occurs when a fetus passes away after the 20th week of pregnancy for the mother. The fetus may have passed away in the uterus days, hours, or even minutes before labor started or even during it.

6. Babies born to overweight or obese moms have an increased risk of being born with heart disease (particularly if you also smoke), developing obesity and overweight as adults, and experiencing other health issues.

Gaining insufficient weight

Lack of weight gain could lead to problems such as early delivery and a child with a low birth weight (less than 2.5kg or 5.5lb at birth). Insufficient fat storage may be the cause.

Your diet and weight before becoming pregnant can have an impact on your ability to acquire weight.

However, some naturally thin women maintain their weight during pregnancy and have healthy offspring.

Controlling pregnancy-related obesity

Pregnant women are now significantly more likely to be obese, and obesity negatively impacts every element of female reproduction. The epidemiological data on pregnancy problems associated with obesity are summarized here. In addition to increased maternal and newborn morbidity and mortality, obesity is associated with several unfavorable obstetric outcomes. Miscarriage, congenital abnormalities, pre-eclampsia, gestational diabetes, Mellitus, iatrogenic preterm birth, postdates pregnancy with higher rates of induction of labor, cesarean section, postpartum hemorrhage, shoulder dystocia, infection, venous thromboembolism, and longer hospital stays are some of these complications. Obese pregnant women must be viewed as a high-risk category with a linear rise in the risk of problems with obesity level.

A multidisciplinary team approach should be used in obstetric management under the direction of consultants to improve outcomes.

Keeping control of your weight growth

It's essential to eat well when you're pregnant to give your child a sound beginning. In any case, you don't need to 'eat for 2', as a few good-natured individuals might have recommended.

You'll most likely find you don't have to consume such a large number of extra kilojoules in the initial 3 months.

A healthy weight increase is expected to result from adding 1,400–1,900 more kilojoules per day in the second and third trimesters as your baby grows. It's perfect to acquire those additional kilojoules from nourishing foods. Fresh fruit and vegetables, wholegrain bread and cereals, legumes, lean meat, fish, and low-fat dairy products are all examples of this.

You ought to make sure that your eating regimen contains the supplements that keep you solid and that will give your child a sound beginning, for example, folic corrosive, iron, calcium, iodine, and protein.

It's essential to stay away from food sources that are high in sugar and added fat and that give no nutrients or minerals.

It's advised that you consume about 2 liters of fluid every day, or more, to maintain your fluid intake. Talk to your doctor or other health care provider if you're not retaining enough fluids because morning sickness can cause dehydration.

The following actions will assist you in gaining the proper amount of weight:

1. Eating a healthy, well-balanced diet that includes fresh fruit and vegetables, whole grain, bread and cereals, legumes, lean meat, fish, and low-fat dairy products, while avoiding fatty and sugary meals and beverages.

2. Exercise regularly, but not too intense

3. Limit your consumption of highly processed, fried, or sugary meals to help you and your unborn child get the proper nutrients.

A nutrient-rich diet not only gives you energy, but also supports your baby's phenomenal growth, which includes the development of her bones, brain, skin, eyes, and digestive system.

Additionally, consuming more protein is necessary for human growth. Your body must also consider the nutrients your kid will need in addition to the protein it needs. For all stages of pregnancy, the RDA advises that pregnant women consume around 1.1 g/kg (0.5 g/lb) of protein. Some academics point out that this sum does not account for the varying needs across the various stages of pregnancy. In early pregnancy (about 16 weeks) and late pregnancy, some will advise consuming 1.2 to 1.52 g/kg (0.5 to 0.7 g/lb) every day (about 36 weeks).

The same holds for women who solely breastfeed.

According to research, you should try to consume 1.7 to 1.9 g/kg (0.8 to 0.09 g/lb) of protein each day to maintain your muscle mass while giving your baby or babies the nutrition they need.

Your daily caloric requirements during pregnancy can benefit from a preliminary estimate. Use your pre-pregnancy calorie intake as a guide for your pregnancy calorie goals, with the daily intake rising each trimester:

First trimester: You probably won't require additional calories yet, except if you began your pregnancy underweight.

Second trimester: Add about an extra 300 to 350 calories each day to your pre-pregnancy diet.

Third trimester: You'll require around 500 calories more each day than you were eating before you got pregnant.

How often should I work out?

You can begin or continue with regular exercise while pregnant, unless your doctor advises otherwise, provided you modify your activity to fit your stage of pregnancy. It will be beneficial to spend about 30 minutes per day walking, swimming, or participating in pregnancy exercise classes. However, you should only engage in 20 minutes of intense exercise at once to prevent overheating.

The best options for exercise during pregnancy are walking, swimming, aqua aerobics, and classes. They'll assist in preventing you from gaining extra weight, maintaining a stable weight (for both normal-weight and obese pregnant women), reducing your weight (for obese pregnant women), lowering your risk of gestational diabetes, and improving your fitness so you can handle labor better.

When pregnant, can you safely lose weight?

The doctor may advise a lady to lose weight if she is extremely overweight before becoming pregnant.

Only with their doctor's supervision should they reduce weight.

The majority of the time, though, pregnant women shouldn't try to diet or lose weight.

How Much Weight to Put On While Pregnant and How Much is Safe

Try these suggestions if your doctor advises weight growth while you are pregnant:

1. Throughout the day, eat five to six small meals.

2. Ensure you always have quick, simple snacks on your hands, such as nuts, raisins, cheese, crackers, dried fruit, ice cream, or yogurt.

3. Toast, crackers, apples, bananas, or lettuce should all be covered in peanut butter. There are around 100 calories and 7 grams of protein in one tablespoon of creamy peanut butter.

4. Mash potatoes, scrambled eggs, and hot cereal can all be made with nonfat powdered milk.

5. Make your food more filling by including extras like cheese, butter or margarine, cream cheese, gravy, sour cream, and so on.

What would you do if you gained too much weight while pregnant?

Assuming that you have put on more weight than your doctor suggested, converse with your doctor about it. The best time to start losing weight is after giving birth.

Here are a few hints to slow your weight gain:

- Choose lower-fat options when eating fast food, such as plain bagels, plain baked potatoes, or a broiled chicken breast sandwich with tomato and lettuce (no sauce or mayonnaise). Steer clear of items like breaded chicken patties, mozzarella sticks, and fries.
- Keep away from entire milk items. You want no less than four servings of milk items consistently. Be that as it may, utilizing skim, 1%, or 2% milk will incredibly diminish how much

calories and fat you eat. Likewise, pick low-fat or without-fat cheese or yogurt.

- Cut back on sugary or sweet beverages. Soft drinks, fruit punch, fruit drinks, iced tea, lemonade, and powdered drink mixes are examples of sweetened beverages that are high in empty calories. To avoid unnecessary calories, choose water, club soda, or mineral water.
- Avoid seasoning food with salt during cooking. You retain water when you consume salt.
- Limit your intake of sugary and caloric snacks. Foods high in calories and low in nourishment include cookies, sweets, doughnuts, cakes, syrup, honey, and potato chips. Avoid consuming these meals daily. As low-

calorie alternatives, consider fresh fruit, low-fat yogurt, angel food cake with strawberries, or pretzels.
- Utilize fats sparingly. Lard, sour cream, cream cheese, gravy, sauces, mayonnaise, ordinary salad dressings, and butter are all examples of fats. Consider less-fat options.
- Healthfully prepare food. When food is fried in oil or butter, calories and fat are added. Boiling, grilling, broiling, and baking are healthier cooking techniques.

Chapter Six
Transform your obese physique into a fit body (prevention and improvement)

While changing your body is admirable, maintaining a fit body and a healthy lifestyle that allow you to enjoy life in a balanced way is much more spectacular.

Fad diets may cause weight reduction, but they rarely help people keep the weight off since you hardly ever develop lifelong healthy habits or alter your perspective on food, exercise, and health.

What to eat

1. Stick to water and avoid consuming too many calorie-dense beverages like alcohol, soda, and juice.

2. Take your time when you eat because if you consume a meal in less than five minutes, there is a good chance that you will consume more food than if you consumed that meal over 30 minutes. This is because your brain needs time to catch up with your stomach before it can detect when you are full.

3. Strive to consume a diet that is high in protein

and low in carbohydrates. It aids in regulating your blood sugar to prevent drastic fluctuations.

4. Consume sufficient amounts of vegetables and limit your intake of fruit, which already contains sugar. Additionally, consume adequate meals high in fiber.

5. Look at the nutrition labels for the number of calories, fat, carbohydrates, and sugar contained in the snack or food you are buying whenever you go shopping. Note: Do not eat foods that contain more than 30-50 grams of carbohydrates and more than 15-25 grams of sugar. A portion of healthy food should have up to 6-7 grams of protein.

6. Eat protein for breakfast.

Numerous diets, pills, and meal replacement programs exist, all of which promise to help you lose weight quickly, but the majority of them are unsupported by any kind of research. But some approaches have scientific support and do help with weight management.

1. Keeping gut bacteria in check:

Focusing on how gut bacteria affect weight management is one new field of study.

Around 37 trillion bacteria are among the numerous and diverse microorganisms that live in the human gut.

Each person's gut contains a unique mix of bacterial species and numbers. Some can boost how much energy a person gets from meals, which can cause fat to accumulate and weight gain.

2. Controlling your level of stress:

As part of the body's fight or flight reaction, stress causes the release of hormones like cortisol and adrenaline, which at first suppress hunger. However, chronic stress can cause cortisol to stay in the system for a longer period, increasing hunger and possibly causing people to eat more. Cortisol alerts the body that it needs to replace its nutritional reserves with its preferred fuel, carbohydrates. The blood's glucose from carbs is subsequently transported by insulin to the muscles and brain. The body will store the sugar as fat if the person does not utilize it during a fight or flight response.

The body mass index (BMI) of children and adolescents who are overweight or obese significantly decreased after the implementation of an 8-week stress-management intervention program, according to research.

Among the techniques for reducing stress are:

Spending time outdoors, such as walking or gardening, practicing yoga, meditation, or tai chi breathing methods

3. A variety of plants:
Eating more fruits, vegetables, and grains will increase fiber absorption and promote a wider range of gut bacterial species. Vegetables and other plant-based foods should make up at least 75% of a person's meal.

4. Fermented foods:
This helps good bacteria perform better while preventing the growth of harmful bacteria. Probiotics are beneficial microorganisms that are found in foods like miso, kimchi, tempeh, kefir, yogurt, and sauerkraut. Kimchi appears to offer anti-obesity properties, according to a large body of research. In a similar vein, research suggests drinking kefir may support weight loss in obese women.

5. Prebiotic foods:
These promote some of the beneficial bacteria's growth and activity, which helps with weight management. Prebiotic fiber can be found in a wide variety of fruits and vegetables

but is particularly abundant in chicory root, artichokes, onions, garlic, asparagus, leeks, bananas, and avocados. Grass foods like oats and barley also contain it.

6. Getting enough sleep each night:

It has been demonstrated in numerous research studies that less than 5 to 6 hours of sleep per night is linked to an increased risk of obesity. There are several causes for this. According to research, getting too little or bad sleep lowers metabolism, the body's process of converting calories into energy. The body may retain extra energy as fat when metabolism is less efficient. A lack of sleep can also lead to a rise in the hormones cortisol and insulin, which promote the storage of fat.

Leptin and ghrelin, two hormones that regulate appetite, are also influenced by how much sleep a person gets. Leptin is responsible for alerting the brain whenever the body feels full.

7. Exercise regularly: Exercise regularly since it is very beneficial for your health. Cardiovascular and strength exercises slow down the functional decline of older people, boost bone density, enhance lean body mass, improve blood and lymphatic circulation, prevent diabetes, reduce visceral fat, and lower blood pressure. Exercise is the highest form of obesity treatment.

8. Exercise or a cold environment can stimulate brown fat tissue. For six weeks, if you spend two hours a day in a room that is 70°C to 62°F below room temperature, you will start to lose some fat.

9. Take regular, 20 to 30-minute walks every day.

10. Research shows that using mental imagery can significantly increase

weight loss. Eight times more weight was lost with Functional Imagery Training (FIT) than with an alternative conversation therapy. The method is made to have people picture how great it will feel to lose weight. Additionally, the imagery exercises assisted persons in reducing their waistlines by roughly two inches. Unexpectedly, neither the participants in the study nor their lifestyles changed in any way. The mental images served just to increase motivation.

11. Portion control is also vital when trying to reduce weight.

12. Increasing physical activity: Although the body burns some calories even when a person is just sitting or sleeping, for most people, the more active

they are, the more calories their bodies will burn. This, however, may take some time. In order for a person to successfully lose one pound of fat, he/she must expend 3,500 calories.

13. Limiting one's exposure to screens, television, and other "sit time"

14. Add more vitamin D to your diet. Several studies show that people with low vitamin D blood levels are more prone to be overweight and engage in insufficient physical activity. Low vitamin D has also been linked to the following health issues: Metabolism Syndrome, Type 1 and Type 2 diabetes, depression, anxiety, osteoporosis, and osteoarthritis. Sunlight and certain foods can provide vitamin D to people. Egg yolks, fatty fish, certain

mushrooms, and foods that have been fortified are examples of foods that contain vitamin D.

How Much Protein Should You Eat Each Day?

The importance of protein for good health cannot be overstated. However, there isn't a set amount of protein that all people should consume daily.

How to ensure that you're getting enough protein for your body is shown here.

The recommended daily intake of protein

It is essential that men and women consume a minimum of 0.8 grams (g) of protein per kilogram (kg) of body weight (or 0.36 g per lb) each day.

Pregnancy, levels of activity, and advanced age are just a few situations where more is necessary.

Additionally, studies correlate weight loss and increased protein consumption. To reduce weight, your protein consumption will therefore vary even more.

How much protein should I consume each day, in grams?

Be aware that when we talk about grams, we mean the grams of the macronutrient protein, not the foods it originates from.

For instance, a large egg only contains slightly more than 6 g of protein despite weighing roughly 50 g.

The current worldwide Recommended Dietary Allowance (RDA) for both men and women is 0.8 grams per kilogram (g/kg) of body weight, or roughly 0.36 grams per pound when it comes to the total quantity of protein you require.

Accordingly, a 150-lb person would need roughly 54 g of protein, but a 200-lb person would require 72 g.

This RDA is the bare minimum to prevent a protein shortage. People who frequently need more protein include:

Athletes: 0.5–0.9 g/lb (1.2–2.0 g/kg).

Ladies who are pregnant: 1.1 g/kg (0.5 g/lb).

1.2 and 2.0 g/kg (0.5-0.9 g/lb) for older persons.

What daily protein intake is recommended for weight loss?

The only macronutrient when it comes to losing weight that never receives a bad rap is protein. The reason is that eating enough protein has been proven to aid in weight loss.

Protein-rich foods have a thermic impact, which speeds up metabolism and increases energy consumption.

Thus, increasing the protein content of your diet may increase energy usage.

In addition to being the most satiating macronutrient, protein also makes you feel full and content after eating.

An after-lunch high-protein snack reduced afternoon hunger, according to a small 2014 study on healthy women.

In comparison to those who ate high-fat, high-carb snacks, 100 fewer calories were ingested at dinner.

It has also been demonstrated that eating more than 1.2 g/kg per day, as opposed to the recommended range of 0.8 to 1.2 g/kg per day, increases feelings of fullness.

Protein should make up 20 to 30 percent of your overall calorie intake to aid in weight loss.

Multiply 0.20 or 0.30 to your daily caloric intake to convert this amount to grams. Next, divide that result by 4 (the number of calories contained per gram of protein).

How much protein should you

consume every day? Let's compute it!

If you are under the age of 65, do not lift weights frequently, are not pregnant, and are not trying to lose weight, then your protein needs may be in line with those of the majority of people at 0.8 g/kg (or 0.36 g/lb) per day.

Take your weight and multiply it by either 0.8 if you're using kilograms or 0.36 if you're using pounds to determine your protein consumption. You will receive the recommended daily intake of protein in grams with this.

The calculation would be as follows, for instance, if you weighed 175 lbs. (or 79 kg): 175 x 0.36 = 63 g OR 79 x 0.8 =

63.2 g

Eat additional protein every day by consuming meals high in it.

The next step is to eat now that you know how many grams of protein you should consume daily.

The top sources of both plant-based and animal-based protein are as follows:

For every 1 oz. of ground beef, there are 7 grams of protein.

Chicken breast has 8 g of protein per 1 oz.

Fish: One ounce of fish has 6 grams of protein.

Eggs provide 6 g of protein per egg.

Vegetables and grains can also satisfy your needs if you're a vegan or vegetarian. Plant-based sources with a high protein content include:

Soy: 3 ounces of firm tofu contain 9 g of protein.

Black beans provide 15 g of protein per cup.

Almonds contains 6 grams of protein per ounce

For every cup of quinoa, there are 8 grams of protein.

Although it's preferable to receive your protein from whole meals, if you find that you're not getting enough, there are various protein powders on the market that can help you catch up.

Pharmacotherapy (pharmacological method) for the Treatment of Obesity

We'll talk about how to treat obesity, so we'll suggest some herbal remedies or medications that help you lose weight and maintain a healthy physique.

Sympathomimetics

The first category of herbs belongs to the stimulant class known as sympathomimetics. It activates the neurological system, raising heart rate, blood pressure, and metabolism as a result. This plant may reduce hunger, but it also occasionally leads to anxiety, insomnia, irritability, a rapid heartbeat, headache, nausea, vomiting, and diarrhea. As soon as you stop taking sibutramine, this symptom disappears.

Orlistat

The second sort of natural treatment is that it contains a craving suppressant called 'orlistat.' It works by impeding the catalyst that your body uses to process fat. As a result, around 25% of the fat you consume is not absorbed by your body. Even when you consume all the calories, orlistat makes you feel full, so you might eat less.

Serotonin

The third category of herbal treatments uses tricyclic, monoamine oxidase, and serotonin reuptake inhibitor (SSRI) antidepressants as well as serotonin reuptake inhibitor (SSRI) antidepressants (MAOI). The way that medications reduce appetite is by telling your brain to quit eating. When you stop taking sibutramine, these side effects disappear. Serotonin can simultaneously treat symptoms including dry mouth, sleepiness, constipation, or diarrhea.

Sibutramine

Two types of diet tablets exist. Ephedrine and caffeine are examples of stimulants in the first category; they raise blood pressure and heart rate. When you stop using sibutramine, these symptoms fade away.

Herbs that impact the body's levels of serotonin make up the second category (the brain chemical that makes you feel good, satisfied, and complete).

Some of these signs, like headaches, nausea, and jitteriness, maybe ones you've heard of. Some persons who experience this symptom may experience severe adverse effects, especially if they also take antidepressants known as monoamine oxidase inhibitors (MAOIs) or selective serotonin reuptake inhibitors (SSRIs).

Herbal remedies for weight loss

Natural medications contrast with regular pharmacological medications. Indeed, spices additionally have nourishing components, and drug fixings associated with polyvalent. At the point when fat transcends normally, it starts to store in different body organs like the liver, muscles, and heart. It creates chemicals and hormones that have a substantial impact on how the body functions. One is more likely to develop ailments associated with obesity if they are overweight or obese. As more individuals become interested in losing weight naturally without using strong drugs and in benefiting from natural herbs, alternative medicine is progressively growing in popularity. Here are a few herbal remedies that can be used to cure obesity.

Ginger (Zingiber officinale):
Ginger has adaptable restorative properties. Large numbers of us know about the mending properties of ginger tea and ginger juice to treat colds. It is effectively accessible in a spice shop.

Antioxidants included in ginger known as gingerols can boost metabolism and elicit a feeling of fullness, which decreases hunger. Additionally, ginger has fat-burning enzymes that aid in the burning of fat, lowering LDL cholesterol and raising HDL cholesterol.

Pepper (Piper nigrum):
Because they benefit your health and appearance in a variety of ways, peppers are arguably one of the most

popular seasonings. Pepper not only contains several anti-aging antioxidants but also has appetite-suppressing qualities that help people lose weight.

Piperine, an ingredient in pepper, improves catechol-O-methyltransferase activity (COMT). Dopamine and norepinephrine are degraded by this enzyme, allowing your body to expel extra fat. White pepper is less helpful in weight loss since this component, which lowers fat levels, is only present in small amounts in black pepper. Thus, black pepper is recommended.

Oregano (Origanum vulgare hirta)

Oregano's potent scent and distinct flavor make it impossible to overlook in meals.

It contains a lot of carvacrol antioxidants, which have potent anti-inflammatory and fat-burning properties.

Oregano not only reduces weight gain but also delays the onset of wrinkles.

Ginseng (Panax ginseng)

For thousands of years, Chinese people have employed ginseng root, which is known for its healing properties. It is often referred to be a natural weight-loss supplement.

Ginseng has ginsenosides, which boost the body's capacity to burn fat cells and suppress appetite. This helps people lose weight by accelerating their metabolism.

Turmeric (Curcuma longa)

In several Asian nations, turmeric—a member of the ginger family—is frequently utilized. Additionally, a lot of individuals utilize turmeric as a remedy for several illnesses, including colds, coughs, and conditions like arthritis and stomachaches.

However, turmeric is a great spice for

weight loss. Turmeric has an antioxidant called curcumin that can reduce fat cells in your body in addition to igniting the enzymatic process that can burn fat and enhance digestion.

Cayenne

Cayenne's primary component, capsaicin, promotes thermogenesis, which can aid in weight loss.

Capsaicin may lessen appetite in addition to boosting metabolism and possibly promoting fat oxidation, which is the body's process of breaking down fat stores.

Fenugreek

There are several ways that fenugreek promotes weight loss. Fenugreek helps people lose weight by releasing insulin and so reducing their hunger. Other supplements, such as hoodia, have been used in conjunction with it.

Honey

Honey can increase the number of calories you burn during the first stages of sleep. Take it right before bed. Essential vitamins, minerals, and good fats are added to this component to make it more nutritious.

Honey contains vital hormones that help with weight loss by reducing appetite.

Obesity treatment at home

Several of the home cures for managing obesity include:

- Keep your stomach full throughout the day by including tomatoes, carrots, and dark leafy vegetables in your diet. These vegetables are beneficial to your health and are minimal in calories.
- One of the best methods for losing weight is drinking green tea. To combat obesity, drink two to three cups of green tea per day.
- Many of us neglect to work out every day. Obesity and being overweight can result from inactivity. Exercise, however, maintains your health and aids in the burning of additional

body fat. Therefore, it's time to start exercising every day.

- One teaspoon of honey and one teaspoon of lemon juice should be combined in a glass of warm water, and this mixture should be consumed every morning.
- Mint leaves are excellent for assisting with weight loss. In the form of peppermint tea, include them in your daily diet. Additionally, you can chew them after meals.
- Body fat can be broken down quickly and effectively using apple cider vinegar. Take 1 teaspoon of lemon juice and 1 teaspoon of apple cider vinegar every day on an empty stomach in a glass of warm water.

Simple exercise instructions
Nowadays, it is well accepted that individuals of all weights who engage in physical

activity are healthier and far less likely to develop chronic diseases.

But the idea of starting any type of exercise regimen might be particularly daunting for the millions of Americans who are classed as obese and who are sedentary — and for good reason. Certain workouts may be too painful or physically uncomfortable for persons who are overweight to accomplish.

The good news is that there are strategies for helping obese, inactive persons ease into a regular exercise regimen so they can benefit from fitness and better health.

Do You Need to Exercise a Lot?

Adults who are overweight or obese should exercise for at least 30 minutes, five days a week or more, at least at a moderate intensity. The task can be completed in a single session or numerous shorter ones lasting 10 minutes or longer.

That may seem like a lot to a newbie who is overweight. But you must consider this suggestion a target toward which you can strive. If you're physically unable to exercise for 30 minutes this week, try your best to increase your time each day until you can. In actuality, three 10-minute workout sessions spread throughout the day result in an equal calorie burn as a continuous 30-minute workout.

Even if your workouts are so brief that they don't add much to the number of calories you burn at first, it doesn't matter. Starting, the only thing that counts is that you're performing to the best of your ability. This is exactly how to get your body ready for lengthier workout sessions in the future.

Even if you split up that 30 minutes into two or three 10- to 15-minute segments spread throughout the day, you'll still reap the rewards of fitness.

Don't let yourself get distracted by the time when you first start. Choose an activity that you will enjoy and can fit into your schedule at least three to five days a week instead.

What sort of workout should you try?

Water aerobics

There are numerous privileges to exercising in the water.

You feel lighter because the water supports your body weight. Additionally, it lessens the strain on your joints, so any discomfort your hips or knees may have from walking on land is essentially nonexistent when you're standing in the water.

Consider signing up for a group exercise session at your neighborhood pool. Additionally, you can consider learning some easy resistance exercises that you can do in the water.

Cycling stationary

The recumbent bike, commonly referred to as a sitting stationary cycle, includes a backrest, making it an ideal option for obese persons. It might be challenging to sit on an upright stationary bike for some obese persons because they lack a strong abdominal core. Another benefit of seated bikes is that they are less demanding on the lower spine, which is a typical complaint among those who are overweight.

Targeting various lower body muscles by combining walking and sitting stationary biking is a wonderful idea.

Movement/dancing

Exercise doesn't need to be structured to be healthy. Put on some music and dance around the home or engage in any other activity that makes you move more quickly. Even a newbie just starting an exercise regimen can walk around for a short while each day.

Conclusion

It's critical to keep in mind that there are no quick remedies for losing weight.

Eating a nourishing diet is the key method to attaining and retaining a healthy weight.

This should consist of 10 portions of fruits and vegetables, whole grains, and high-quality protein.

Exercising for at least 30 minutes each day is also advantageous.

Both adults and children can be obese (BMI over 30). Shortness of breath, exhaustion and joint discomfort are a few of the symptoms it produces. Due to societal stigma, obesity can also result in psychological issues including depression and low self-esteem. Obesity frequently coexists with medical disorders such as asthma, diabetes, and high blood pressure. Heart issues, strokes, and kidney illness are examples of complications.

Over the past 30 years, obesity rates have risen globally. Changes in government and health care system policies are required to effectively address the issue. The Obesity settle's main focus is education, which is essential even if insufficient on its own.

The fact that no system will take responsibility is the biggest barrier to combating the obesity pandemic. Obese people are solely to blame, according to doctors, the insurance sector, food producers, and the US government. Most individuals consider being overweight to be a severe character fault or a lack of ability to make wise decisions. The personal responsibility paradigm, however, appears to be flawed, according to data, especially that which relates to childhood obesity in youngsters who aren't able to make such decisions.

The food sector bears a large portion of the blame. Scientific experts as well as government organizations in the United States have long promoted the myths that all calories are created equal and that calories are the basis of nutrition. During that period, the sugar industry invaded virtually every category of processed food on the market, adding sweetener to foods that didn't require it while demonizing fat, which is generally safe. The United States Department of Agriculture is one of the federal organizations that helped to codify these beliefs.

People can only reject or withstand highly processed foods to a considerably lesser extent than is commonly believed, especially refined sugar. Sugar addiction exists. Like other addictive substances, eating a lot of it alters the brain's hedonic circuits. It becomes more difficult to enjoy eating healthy food the more sugar a person consumes. Consuming refined sugar causes an insulin surge that causes the body to suffer greatly. Leptin, a hormone that regulates hunger, and ghrelin, a hormone that regulates fullness, both have issues when the body is subjected to excessive insulin. High cortisol levels in the body, which are related to the chronic stress of the modern lifestyle, exacerbate these problems.